The Plant-Based Diet Meal Plan

A New Complete 4 Weeks Vegetarian Meal Plan, with Delicious Recipes, to lose up to 20 Pounds in 30 Days

Vegetarian Academy

© Copyright 2021 by Vegetarian Academy - All rights reserved.

The following Book is reproduced below with the goal of providing information that is as accurate and reliable as possible. Regardless, purchasing this Book can be seen as consent to the fact that both the publisher and the author of this book are in no way experts on the topics discussed within and that any recommendations or suggestions that are made herein are for entertainment purposes only. Professionals should be consulted as needed prior to undertaking any of the action endorsed herein.

This declaration is deemed fair and valid by both the American Bar Association and the Committee of Publishers Association and is legally binding throughout the United States.

Furthermore, the transmission, duplication, or reproduction of any of the following work including specific information will be considered an illegal act irrespective of if it is done electronically or in print. This extends to creating a secondary or tertiary copy of the work or a recorded copy and is only allowed with the express written consent from the Publisher. All additional right reserved.

The information in the following pages is broadly considered a truthful and accurate account of facts and as such, any inattention, use, or misuse of the information in question by the reader will render any resulting actions solely under their purview. There are no scenarios in which the publisher or the original author of this work can be in any fashion deemed liable for any hardship or damages that may befall them after undertaking information described herein.

Additionally, the information in the following pages is intended only for informational purposes and should thus be thought of as universal. As befitting its nature, it is presented without assurance regarding its prolonged validity or interim quality. Trademarks that are mentioned are done without written consent and can in no way be considered an endorsement from the trademark holder.

Tables of Contents

INTRODUCTION 6
CALORIES TABLES AND DESCRIPTION OF PLANT-BASED FOODS AND MICRONUTRIENTS 10
THE PLANT-BASED DIET MEAL PLAN (STARTING MEAL PLAN) 17
    PLANNING THE PLANT-BASED MEAL 23
THE PLANT-BASED DIET MEAL PLAN 30
    WEEK 1 32
    WEEK 2 38
    WEEK 3 45
    WEEK 4 50

THE PLANT BASED BREAKFAST 56
    CHIA FLAXSEED WAFFLES 56
    CAULIFLOWER ZUCCHINI FRITTERS 58
    CHOCOLATE STRAWBERRY MILKSHAKE 60
    COCONUT BLACKBERRY BREAKFAST BOWL 62
    CINNAMON COCONUT PANCAKE 64
    FLAX ALMOND MUFFINS 66
    GRAIN-FREE OVERNIGHT OATS 68
    ZUCCHINI MUFFINS 70
    APPLE AVOCADO COCONUT SMOOTHIE 72
    HEALTHY BREAKFAST GRANOLA 73
    CHIA CINNAMON SMOOTHIE 75
    VEGETABLE TOFU SCRAMBLE 76

THE PLANT BASED LUNCH 78
    MAC & "CHEESE" 78
    THAI SQUASH SOUP 80
    BUTTER BEAN HUMMUS 82
    SPINACH & ORANGE SALAD 84
    LENTIL & SWEET POTATO SOUP 86
    FRUITY KALE SALAD 88
    BLACK EYED PEAS STEW 90
    WHITE BEAN & SPINACH SOUP 91

SOUP SALADS AND SIDES 93

THE PLANT-BASED DIET MEAL PLAN

Mexican Cauliflower Rice 93
Turnip Salad 95
Brussels sprouts Salad 96
Tomato Eggplant Spinach Salad 97
Cauliflower Radish Salad 100
Celery Salad 102
Ginger Avocado Kale Salad 103
Avocado Cabbage Salad 105
Vegetable Salad 106
Refreshing Cucumber Salad 108
Avocado Almond Cabbage Salad 109

Introduction

Plant-based weight control plans offer all the essential protein, fats, carbohydrates, nutrients, and minerals for ideal wellbeing, and are regularly higher in fiber and phytonutrients. Notwithstanding, a few vegans may need to include an enhancement (explicitly nutrient B12) to guarantee they get every one of the nutrients required.

There is no reasonable meaning of what comprises an entire nourishment, plant-based eating regimen (WFPB diet). The WFPB diet isn't really a set eating regimen — it's to a greater degree a way of life. This is on the grounds that plant-based eating regimens can shift enormously relying upon the degree to which an individual incorporates creature items in their eating regimen.

Regardless, the essential standards of an entire nourishments, plant-based diet are as per the following:

Emphasizes entire, negligibly handled nourishments.

Limits or stays away from creature items.

Excludes refined nourishments, as included sugars, white flour and handled oils.

Pays extraordinary consideration regarding nourishment quality, with numerous advocates of the WFPB diet advancing privately sourced, natural nourishment at whatever point conceivable.

Hence, this eating regimen is regularly mistaken for vegan or vegetarian eats less. However, albeit comparable here and there, these weight control plans are not the equivalent.

For all the vegetarians and plant lovers, there is a plant-based diet plan available that helps them to get better and in good shape. The new form of vegetarian diet helps the people to look great, stay active and be healthy. It is an all plant and no meat diet that is easy to digest, fresh and gives numerous benefits as well.

Normally, people consider that plants come with limited options but in reality, it is very different. For a hardcore plant-based food plan there are numerous options available for a person. These ground growing food items have numerous nutrition, vitamins and other resources in them that are not measurable. If a person is good enough to prepare a list of ultimate food options and get the right guide for the plant-based diet, they will get maximum benefit.

Here in this book, you can find everything you need to know about the plant-based diet. From its basics to the ultimate diet plans and recipes there is everything available of your interest. It is a composite and complete resource for you that help you to follow the diet plan in all healthy manners and take full advantage of it. All you need is to go through these resources and manage everything as per your own preferences.

People have over time managed to interpret plant-based meals to other products that are inclusive of meat in the diet. That remains a controversy as different cultures have different beliefs. The rise of processed foods over the years has brought deceases and other challenges in the food industry. This is the reason why a good number of individuals have decided to turn to plant-based meals as they believe it reduces the chances of diseases and well as it being cost-effective in one way or another. People will argue that there is no difference in a full meal diet and a plant-based meal, but science has proven that they are indeed different.

Plant-based meals are considered to be healthier as compared to other types of meals. Fast food is the order of the day as the human race has become so busy to even take a look on their health meaning that it is possible for a large population to have grown far away from healthy living. This book emphasizes the importance of a healthy lifestyle as well as gives instructions on how to change and start on the journey of healthy living by incorporating a plant-based meal in each and everyone's meal plans. By choosing a healthy lifestyle, a person will be able to be in control of their body fat content and also check their weight as this will be more beneficial to them in a healthy way and guarantee them a life that is less of strange diseases with lots of expenses on drugs and checkups.

Calories Tables And Description Of Plant-based Foods And Micronutrients

Plants are rich in micronutrients that come from the soil they grow in, the basics of life they need to grow, the phytochemicals they use to protect themselves, attract insects and adapt to the changes around them. As plants are unable to move as animals do, they have a uniquely full tool chest of macro and micro-nutrients that enable them to adapt to the changing environment around them. These micronutrients are just as valuable to humans as they are to the plants but in different ways. Below is a breakdown of the basic micronutrients found in fruits, vegetables, nuts, seeds, and legumes.

Vitamins
Vibrant vegetables and fruits are a dense source of vitamins that are essential to overall health and wellness.

Vitamin A: Also known as beta-carotene is a carotenoid found in yellow, orange and dark green fruits and veg, most notably carrots, spinach, and broccoli. It protects against infections and is essential for eye and skin health.

Vitamin B: This group of vitamins is responsible for maintaining the nervous system and cognitive function, DNA and blood cell production.

1 is responsible for nervous system health and aids in the breakdown and absorption of food. Found in peas, whole grains, and most fruits and vegetables.

2 is responsible for energy production and healthy skin and eyes and found in asparagus, spinach, and broccoli.

3 is great for healthy skin and energy production and is found in peanuts, avocados, peas, and mushrooms.

6 is also essential for energy production and is found in chickpeas, potatoes, banana, squash, and nuts.

9 is also known as folate and is essential for fetal development and growth and healthy cell division. It is found in legumes, asparagus, spinach, arugula, kale, and beets.

12 is predominantly sourced from animal products but you can find it in some organic soy products but most notably nutritional yeast.

Vitamin C: An essential vitamin important for cell growth and energy production as well as tissue repair and wound healing. It is one of the most powerful antioxidants and is found in strawberries, spinach, Brussel sprouts, sweet potatoes, and tomatoes.

Vitamin E: A powerful antioxidant that protects the body from free radical damage including premature aging. It's of great support to the immune system, protecting it against external pathogens. It is found in sunflower seeds, almonds, hazelnuts, spinach, and broccoli.

Vitamin K: This vitamin plays a major role in the clotting cascade and also in bone health. It is found in all green leafy veg as well as cruciferous veg and green tea.

Minerals

Macro-minerals: we need these in large quantities from our diet.

Calcium: This essential mineral plays roles in bone, heart, muscle and nerve health. Foods high in calcium are spinach, collard greens, seeds, almonds, soybeans, and butter beans.

Chloride: This mineral plays a part in body fluid balance including digestive juices. It is found in sea salt, tomatoes, lettuce, celery, and rye bread.

Magnesium: This mineral regulates blood sugar and assists in energy production. It also helps your muscles, kidneys, bones and heart function effectively. It is found in spinach, quinoa, dark chocolate, almonds, avocado, and black beans.

Phosphorous: This mineral is found in bones and works with calcium in maintaining healthy mineral balance within the body. It is found in pumpkin, sunflower seeds, lentils, chickpeas, oatmeal, and quinoa.

Sodium: The current population gets excess sodium from all pre-packaged foods and restaurant meals, so there is no need to go looking for extra sodium in the diet.

Potassium: This mineral is essential in blood pressure balance, muscle health, and nerve function. It is found in avocado, bananas, apricots, grapefruit, potatoes, mushrooms, cucumbers and zucchini.

Trace Minerals

We just need tiny amounts of these from our foods.

Copper: Essential in the formation of red blood cells and iron absorption. It is found in whole grains, beans, potatoes, cocoa, black pepper, and dark leafy greens.

Cobalt: This trace mineral works closely with B12 in the formation of hemoglobin. It is found in nuts, broccoli, oats, and spinach.

Manganese: Plays many roles in enzyme activity and cellular level antioxidants. It is found in pineapple, peanuts, brown rice, spinach, sweet potato, pecans, and green tea.

Iodine: Essential for thyroid function, you can find it in seaweed, lima beans, and prunes.

Iron: Used to make hemoglobin and as a carrier for essential nutrients in the blood. In plant form, it is found in cashews, spinach, whole grains, tofu, potatoes, and lentils.

Selenium: A trace mineral essential in the role of reproduction, DNA production, and antioxidant function. It is found in brazil nuts, lentils, cashew nuts, and potatoes.

Zinc: As your body doesn't store zinc, it needs to be consumed daily because it plays important roles in nutrient metabolism, immune system maintenance, and enzyme function. It is found in legumes, nuts, seeds, potatoes, kale and green beans.

Colors

The colors in fruits and vegetables point to what kinds of nutrients they contain.

White foods: Contain sulfur and can have anti-cancer properties. Found in cauliflower, garlic, leeks, and onions.

Green foods: Contain lutein and vitamin K. Found in dark leafy greens, broccoli, avocado.

Purple foods: Contain anthocyanins, which are powerful antioxidants. Found in blueberries, eggplant, red cabbage, and blackberries.

Red foods: Contain lycopene and has therapeutic properties for the heart. Found in strawberries, watermelon, tomatoes, and red bell peppers.

The Plant-based Diet Meal Plan (starting Meal Plan)

Plant-based meal arranging is somewhat more confused in the first place contrasted with simply preparing up arbitrary meals. Things being what they are, the reason the hell would it be a good idea for you to try and trouble and instruct yourself on the best way to meal plan appropriately? All things considered, it can offer you a larger number of advantages than you may suspect.

How Would You Like:

A complain free week

Less basic leadership and overthinking meals

Easier shopping and a lower grocery bill

Effortlessly adhering to sound propensities

Easily meeting individual healthful needs

Trying new recipes

Having an arrangement for your weight loss or weight gain

Knowing what works best for you

Keeping yourself responsible by having every one of the fixings and meals close by

Beginning Tips

Before we're getting directly into the vegan meat of the issue, there are a couple of tips to think about that can make your meal arranging venture significantly simpler, less startling, and substantially more energizing! We truly need you to succeed and this implies you're getting a charge out of the procedure just as the outcomes here. Step by step instructions to Do It

Try not to Spend All Day on Meal Prepping

Except if you need to get worn out or meal prep is your obsession. Pull out all the stops! Something else, set a clock for two hours and when it dings you are DONE! That is sufficient opportunity to prep veggies, vegetables, cook grains, and select recipes if necessary. Make the most of your end of the week! Try not to do a lot without a moment's delay. You'll be astounded at what you can achieve in two centered hours.

Make An Arrangement

Put aside 45 minutes or thereabouts and select your recipes for the week. Spare them on your telephone by taking a screen capture or spare them on a Pinterest board or go old fashioned and print them out! Simply keep them somewhere sheltered! This guide allows you 30 days of recipes for breakfast, lunch, and dinner, so you have the opportunity to build up a framework that works for you going ahead!

Set aside Cash

Shop the deals in the Sunday paper. (Truly, this is as yet a thing!) Select your week by week recipes as indicated by what you can purchase for less! Verify what grocery stores in your general vicinity twofold coupons. You can spare a TON along these lines and no; you don't need to be an outrageous coupon to do it! Spare huge internet shopping by utilizing applications like Ebates and ibotta. Their costs are up to half off – everyday – and – they convey!

Use Multi-Purpose Recipes

Discover recipes you can twofold or you realize will consider scraps you can have for lunch. You know, Monday night's bean stew transforms into Tuesday's Taco sort of thing! I've incorporated a few multi-reason plant-based recipes beneath on the off chance that you're intrigued. See bean stew, soups, and [vegan] burgers.

Cluster Cook

Concoct a major cluster of entire grains like dark colored rice, quinoa, or grain to go with your week by week meals on Saturday or Sunday. Douse and cook chickpeas and beans on your favored meal prep day. At that point portion them out for plates of mixed greens, buddha bowls, and bean stews. This procedure won't take up your whole day, yet it will spare you huge amounts of time later in the week!

Try not to Get Too Gourmet

Start with straightforward recipes and develop your direction. Start with simple recipes!

Picking Your Food

There are a lot of interesting points when picking the nourishments which you will incorporate into your meal plan. Once more, remember these to make the procedure progressively charming and fun! Along these lines, for your plant-based meal arranging, ensure you...

Go for the nourishments you effectively like before purchasing an immense sack of Brussel's sprouts or rhubarb

Use what you have at home to set aside cash and abstain from squandering any nourishment

Keep a running rundown of what you need so you won't overlook anything and remain well-supplied

Make a grocery rundown to go out on the town to shop each week

Go for mass areas and occasional produce to set aside some cash

Look out for solidified or pre-cut/pre-destroyed produce and canned vegetables to make your life simpler

Next, stock up your kitchen! By what other methods would you have the option to browse a decent assortment of delicious, solid, and adaptable nourishments to use in your meal plan?

Additional tip: Have an unfaltering stock of snacks in the house, for example, fruit, nuts, and wafers!

Planning The Plant-based Meal

Since you've found out about the absolute most significant establishments, we can get into the arranging it-hard and fast part. When thinking of an idea for a meal plan, we like to concentrate on the accompanying rules. Check whether your nourishment or meals are:

Nutrient thick

Low in included fat, salt and sugar

Rich in fiber

Filling and fulfilling

Based on starches

Adequate to meet your caloric and nourishing needs

This may appear to be somewhat unique to you at the present time, so we needed to give you an understanding of what your meals ought to resemble. When taking a gander at the distinctive nourishment classes, here are the means by which you could make sweet or flavorful balanced vegan meals.

Breakfast Blueprint

Pick at least one of every classification - for cutting edge plant munchers, don't hesitate to include a few vegetables like spinach or solidified cauliflower to your smoothies.

Starches

Oats, bread, grain, hash tans, flapjacks

Fruit

New, dried, solidified, for example, berries, apples, bananas

Vegetables

Soy milk, soy yogurt, tofu (for scramble), nutty spread

Nuts and Seeds

Flaxseeds, chia seeds, pecans, almond spread

Lunch and Dinner Blueprint

Once more, pick one or a few instances of every class - relying upon your vitality or weight objectives, you can join more vegetables or nuts.

Additional items

Nuts, seeds, nut or seed margarine, fruit, sauces, spices, condiments

With respect to snacks, there are no fixed principles – simply do whatever it takes not to utilize this season of day to sneak some garbage or candy machine nourishment into your eating regimen. Some better thoughts are crisp fruit, dried fruit, nuts, entire grain wafers, rice cakes, hummus, veggie sticks, cooked chickpeas, granola bars, sans oil popcorn, or just a few scraps.

You may be thinking now: "Yet in what capacity will I meet the entirety of my wholesome needs on the off chance that I don't generally follow my nourishment? Isn't that difficult on a plant-based eating routine?" This next part is for you to teach yourself and facilitate your brain.

Nutrients and Foods to Focus On

It is great to begin by saying that an entire nourishments plant-based eating routine is just about the most nutrient-thick diet you could think of. That being stated, there are still approaches to pass up a couple of basic ones in the event that you don't concentrate on a decent assortment of nourishments. A few people like to simply eat a lot of fruit or starches, overlooking vegetables and seeds for instance.

It's not actually simpler for individuals on an omnivorous eating routine to meet the entirety of their wholesome needs since they normally get too little fiber, nutrients, and minerals while having an excess of immersed fat and cholesterol. In this way, everybody ought to design their eating regimen astutely!

Concerning the couple of nutrients that are somewhat harder to jump on an absolutely plant-based eating routine, here are the best sources to go for and incorporate into your everyday diet. Pick in any event one for every nutrient:

Calcium: strengthened soy milk, tofu, kale, broccoli, vegetables, sesame, entire wheat

Iron: vegetables, tofu, tomato sauce, dull green vegetables, oats, quinoa, darker rice

Zinc: pumpkin seeds, vegetables, entire grains, verdant green vegetables

Omega-3: flaxseed, chia seeds, pecans, romaine lettuce

Vitamin B12: supplements, strengthened nourishment

Vitamin D: daylight, a few mushrooms, strengthened nourishments, supplements

Portions and Calories

You may even now be pondering about the amount to eat on a plant-based eating regimen. In case you're not mindful of your everyday suggested vitality consumption, check your BMR and include your movement level utilizing a straightforward number cruncher. Most adults need around at any rate 2000 calories for every day which you shouldn't attempt to undermine excessively, in any event, when attempting to get in shape.

Plant-based nourishments, particularly when entire and natural, have a lower calorie thickness which means you should eat bigger portions and it will be significantly simpler to lose some weight in light of the fact that these nourishments include considerably more mass.

If you wind up excessively stuffed or too hungry following a day of eating, make a note and modify in like manner the following day or at whatever point you're making your new meal plan. We can't disclose to you precisely the amount you have to eat, so please have your age, sex, action level, anxiety, and wellbeing status at the top of the priority list. We're advocates for eating naturally, which means go get something when you're ravenous and quit chomping when you're easily full. It's on you to choose what number of meals every day you'd like to eat and if you need to snack. Various things work for various individuals here. Regardless of if it's 2, 3, 4, or 5 little meals for each day – work with your inclinations and your calendar.

Redoing for Weight Goals

When altering your meal plan to your needs and objectives, we prompt that you move your concentration starting with one nutrition type then onto the next and not to remove something totally. All entire plant-based nourishments are gainful to your wellbeing (insofar as you're not prejudiced or oversensitive to them) and can be eaten. We're working with the guideline of calorie thickness here which you can use to either lose, gain, or keep up your weight while powering your body with sound nourishments.

In case you're into weight picking up or lifting weights, center more around entire flour items and vegetables just as nuts, seeds, and dried fruit to get enough calories.

The equivalent goes for individuals with a little craving who battle with eating enough. You may likewise need to incorporate more smoothies and even squeezes into your eating routine to build your calories. Go simple on enormous crude servings of mixed greens and vegetable stews since they offer just barely any calories while including a great deal of mass. Similarly, in case you're into weight loss, center around non-boring vegetables to go with your entire, flawless starches like potatoes or dark colored rice for lunch and dinner. Try not to decrease the starches excessively, have around half vegetables and starches on your plate. Go simple on flour items and dried fruit, have crisp fruit as a snack and attempt to eat a green serving of mixed greens each day. Likewise, keep away from included oils and lessen the measure of nuts and seeds you devour.

The Plant-based Diet Meal Plan

In contrary to the popular belief, transitioning to a plant-based diet is quite easy, if you take the right steps at the right time. By switching to a diet that includes more fibers, vitamins and minerals and avoiding meat and dairy products, you are not depriving yourself from any necessary nutrients. In fact, you are taking a step towards health improvement and a better life in general. Following this 4-week program for transitioning to a plant-based diet will get you the results you wanted, which are healthy eating habits and the ability to enjoy food like you always did.

What is important to know when starting to transition to a plant-based diet is that this process should be done gradually. You should by no means drop meat and dairy ingredients right away and strictly force yourself to eat plant-based foods. The point of this program is to make your transition easy and effortless by gradually creating habits that are going to lead to a full transition without craving to return to your old eating habits. So, take it easy, step by step, and let's get into it!

Week 1

At the very beginning of your transition journey, you are going to start learning which foods to turn to and which ingredients to leave behind. The key here is to take things slowly, which is why in the first week you should focus on your breakfasts. Your meal plan for this week is going to consist of your regular meals with a bit of adjustments done to them. As this is the first stage of your plant-based diet transition process, you need to start balancing your usual diet with the changes you are about to introduce to it. For the beginning, go through the contents of your refrigerator and try to take out as many animal products as possible. Stock your refrigerator with plant-based ingredients to start your transition process! Foods you should be bringing into your fridge include berries, cabbage, broccoli, kale, beans, etc. Also, when choosing your ingredients, look for good quality and check the origin of the products, as you don't want anything processed to find a way to your kitchen.

Don't feel like you need to start avoiding meat and other animal foods right away. There should be no pressure to do so, as this is a calm and slow diet transition. In week 1 we are going to attack your breakfast habits while the rest of your meals of the day are going to stay the same. To help prepare yourself for the second week of your transition process, try to balance your plate by adding more plant-based ingredients than you used to. The more you increase your whole foods intake at this stage of the transition, the easier it is going to be to adjust to what the second, third and fourth week has to offer! Therefore, in week 1, your goal is to switch to plant-based breakfasts with fiber and high nutritional value. Here are three breakfast recipes for you to get inspired to start changing your morning meal habits.

#1 Three Minutes Oatmeal

Ingredients:
- 1/2 cup of oats
- 1 ripe banana
- 1 teaspoon of cinnamon
- 1 teaspoon of grounded flax seeds
- ½ cup of water
- ½ cup of plant-based milk (soy/ rice/ almond/ hemp)

- Toppings of choice (peanut butter/ fresh fruit/ frozen berries/ seeds/ nuts)

Directions:

Roast the oats, flax seeds together with cinnamon on a preheated non-stick pan for about 30 seconds. Add water and milk - start with little and rather add more to reach your desired consistency. Shortly before finishing, add sliced ripe banana (spotted), that is going to serve as a substitute for a sweetener.

Use this recipe as a base on how to prepare oatmeal and try to experiment with other ingredients such as frozen berries, nut butter, cacao, spices (turmeric), nuts or seeds. Mix those ingredients into the oatmeal either while cooking or only when serving as a topping.

Remember that you are trying to avoid processed foods. Therefore, do not forget to read the labels when purchasing your ingredients. Peanut butter should have only one ingredient - peanuts. You do not want any added salt, oil or sugar. The same is valid for dried fruits and plant-based milk (avoid added sugar). It is simple, just read the ingredients of the products.

#2 Overnight Oats

Ingredients:
- ½ cup of oats
- ½ cup of nuts or seeds of choice (walnuts, hazelnuts, sunflower seeds, pumpkin seeds, ...)
- Dried fruit of choice (resins, cranberries, dates)

Directions:

Do you want to prepare your breakfast the night before and not lose time in the morning? Just mix all the ingredients together and simply soak them overnight. In the morning just pour the excess water away and breakfast is served. If desired you can add some fresh fruit.

Soaking oats, nuts and seeds makes them easier digestible. It also wakes up a different taste in them, that you might have not experienced before.

#3 Green Smoothie

Smoothie is a good breakfast when you want to start your day quickly and right away with a bunch of nutrients. The beauty of a smoothie is that you can add ingredients that you otherwise have problems adding to your diet. Perfect examples are greens such as spinach or kale.

For beginners, green smoothies might be quite a challenge. Therefore, I recommend starting with adding just a small portion of greens and slowly increase the amount over time as you get used to the taste.

Generally, the best basis for a smoothie are bananas as they make the smoothie nicely thick and naturally sweet. Always make sure that your fruits are ripe as fruit in that form is the easiest to digest. Ripe bananas are easy to recognize - the color is yellow (not green) with black spots.

Ingredients:

- 2 ripe bananas
- 1 cup fresh baby spinach
- 1 cup frozen berries
- 1 cup of water or plant-based milk

Directions:

First fill the blender with greens, then bananas or other fruits of your choice and liquid (water or plant-based milk). Blend until smooth.

Week 2

In the second week of your transition to a plant-based diet you should be used to eating whole foods and plant-based ingredients for breakfast. Now we are going to step things up and introduce those ingredients to your lunch meals. Therefore, the second week of the program is going to consist of both breakfast and lunch meals made without animal products or any kinds of processed ingredients. You should focus on eliminating dairy products from your lunch meals as well as in general. There's no need to worry about calcium and other nutrients necessary for bone health, as you can get those from healthier plant-based sources as well.

As the second week progresses, you will start learning how to effectively plan your meals and stay on track with your meal plans throughout the week. Dedicate a few minutes every Sunday to creating a meal plan for the following week. This way, you won't run out of ideas for breakfast, lunch or dinner for each day of the week. However, for now, we are only focusing on breakfast and lunch. Therefore, prepare to ditch animal food and combine plant-based ingredients into your lunch meals as well! Here are three recipes to get you started.

#1 Tortilla Pizza

Ingredients:
- Tortilla (optimally wholegrain)
- Tomato sauce or tomato paste
- Vegetable of choice as toppings (suggestion: sliced tomato, corn, garlic, red onion, ...)
- Herbs and spices (oregano, garlic powder)
- Nutritional yeast (optional)

Directions:
Preheat your oven to 200°C.

If you are using bought tomato sauce then, as always, don't forget to check the ingredients. Make sure the sauce is not high in salt (the salt intake should not exceed 1 gram for 100 gram of the sauce) and that all ingredients are plant based: no cheese, meat or eggs.

If you decided to make your own sauce, also check the package of the tomato paste for the salt intake. Place the paste on a pan and add a little bit of water as the paste itself is thick already. When using this sauce for pizza I would recommend keeping it rather thicker. However, you can use the same sauce as a pasta sauce. In that case water it down. Add a teaspoon of dried oregano and a teaspoon of garlic powder. You might also want to add some chili if you prefer spicy food. If you want to add a bit of cheesy flavor to the sauce mix in also a tablespoon of nutritional yeast. You can also sprinkle the whole pizza with nutritional yeast once it is ready to be baked.

As your sauce is ready, spread it on a tortilla like you would do on a pizza dough. Now is the time to get creative with your favorite pizza toppings. If you want to top it with basil leaves or some greens, I recommend doing so only after the baking process as the leaves would burn in the oven.

To bake your pizza faster, and for more crunchy results, do not use baking tin and only bake the pizza on the grate.

Lower the temperature of the oven to 180°C and bake the pizza for approximately 15 minutes until the crust turns brown.

#2 Baked Sweet Potatoes with Avocado-Beans salad

Ingredients:
- 1 big or 2 small sweet potatoes
- ½ of an avocado
- ½ can of red beans
- 1 cup fresh spinach
- 1 tomato
- Pepper, salt (optional)

Directions:
Preheat the oven to 250°C. Wash the sweet potatoes and poke a few holes in them using a knife to fasten the baking process. Place the potatoes on a baking paper in the oven, lower the temperature to 200°C and bake for about 40 to 60 minutes. The baking time is always dependent on your oven. Sweet potatoes are fully baked once sugar is running out of them and they are fork tender.

Meanwhile you have time to prepare your filling. Mash one half of an avocado in a bowl, add beans, diced tomato, pepper (freshly grounded if possible) and optionally salt and mix it all together. In general, try to slowly leave out salt from your diet - especially table salt. Don't worry; your taste buds quickly adapt to new tastes and you will not miss added salt in your meals after a short period of time. If you are not ready to leave out table salt out of your diet, substitute it rather with sea salt or pink Himalayan salt.

Once the potatoes are baked, cut them open. Mash the inside with a fork and create space for the filling. Add spinach leaves first and the avocado mixture on the top. Enjoy!

As with every dish in this book, try not to get stuck with a certain recipe. I would like to give you a guideline for the beginning. Moreover, I would like to encourage you to be creative. Nobody says you cannot add paprika next time instead of tomato, chickpeas instead of red beans or hummus instead of avocado. Remember you are adapting a new lifestyle, not just dieting for 4 weeks.

#3 Red Lentil Soup

Ingredients:
- 1 cup red lentils
- 4 cups of water or low- sodium veggie broth
- 1 table spoon olive oil
- 1 large carrot (diced)
- 1 large onion (diced)
- 1 ½ teaspoon of grounded cardamom
- ½ teaspoon of salt
- Black pepper
- Juice of 1 lemon

Directions:

Heat olive oil in a big pot. Add onion and cardamom, salt and little bit of black pepper and stir until the onion turns little brown. Add lentils and carrots and stir to combine. In this time, the soup is getting its most flavor, so spend a few minutes constantly mixing it, so it doesn't burn at the bottom.

Finally add water or veggie broth (4 cups for each cup of lentils), cover the pot and let it cook on low heat for about 15- 20 minutes.

How do you recognize if it's done? Firstly, when tasting the lentils. Red lentils are falling apart while cooking. Therefore, they should be melting in your mouth when tasting. Secondly, check the carrots with stabbing a piece with a knife. Once the piece slides down the knife, the carrot is cooked. In case it sticks on the knife, keep cooking. This rule generally counts for coking any kind of root vegetable.

When finished cooking, add freshly squeezed lemon juice. Mix it all in and enjoy.

You can keep the soup refrigerated for 5 days. However, it is going to thicken with every day, so you can either water it down or keep it as it is and use it as sauce to be eaten with rice, couscous, quinoa or bread.

Are you enjoying the recipes so far?

Week 3

In week three you are going to switch your dinner meals to the plant-based diet, that is, use only plant-based ingredients to prepare your food. With the third week, you are already wrapping up the transition, as you are now used to your new breakfast and lunch meal strategies. All it takes now is to start implementing those strategies to your dinner meals. At this point, you should already be feeling the improvement in your life caused by starting to transition to a plant-based diet.

With numerous recipes and tips, making plant-based meals is quick and easy, yet as delicious and healthy as you can imagine! In your week three of the transition process you are already near the end of it. What's left to do is introduce these changes to your dinner meals as well and in that way, wrap up a completely new meal plan you are going to be creating every Sunday to stay on track with what you're eating! Here are some delicious and easy plant-based dinner recipes!

#1 Bulgur Salad

Ingredients:
- ½ cup bulgur wheat
- Diced vegetable of your choice (paprika, celery, tomatoes)
- ½ cup chickpeas
- 1 cup spinach (diced)
- ½ avocado
- Pepper, salt, oregano, powdered garlic

Directions:

There are two options how to prepare bulgur. If you need to prepare your dish quickly, then simply cook bulgur (1 cup bulgur for 2 cups cold water) in a pot. Bring to a boil, cover the pot and let simmer for 12-15 minutes until tender.

Another option is to soak the bulgur before. Ideally, overnight, but already an hour is enough. Strain it afterwards, rinse one more time and you're good to go. The soaked version tastes lighter and refreshing.

Mash an avocado in a bowl and combine with bulgur. Add in chickpeas and prepared vegetables diced on small pieces. Finally add in seasonings according to your taste. Give it a final mix and enjoy!

#2 Almond noodles

Ingredients:
- 100 g of whole grain spaghetti
- ½ cup of almond butter
- ¼ cup of water
- ¼ cup of rice vinegar
- 2 tablespoons of low sodium soy sauce or tamari
- 2 tablespoons of Thai red curry paste
- Chopped fresh cilantro
-

Directions:
To prepare this nutrient rich and flavorful dish, cook the spaghetti as you regularly would, while, in the meantime, mix the almond butter, rice vinegar, water, soy sauce or tamari and the Thai red curry paste and whisk it together in a large bowl. Once the spaghetti is cooked, add it into the sauce and mix it together. Serve the meal with the chopped cilantro on top and enjoy!

#3 Pumpkin Soup

Ingredients:
- 500 g pumpkin (without seeds)
- 3 cloves garlic (unpeeled)
- 1 table spoon olive oil
- Pepper (amount depending on your own taste)
- ½ teaspoon Turmeric
- Salt (optional)
- Cayenne pepper, chili (optional)
- Boiled water or low- sodium veggie broth

Directions:

Preheat your oven to 200°C.

Remove the pumpkin seeds and cut the pumpkin to pieces about 2 inches big. Mix them in a bowl together with garlic cloves, olive oil, pepper, turmeric, salt if needed and if you like spicy food you can also add cayenne pepper or chili powder.

Spread prepared pumpkin on a baking tin with baking sheet (moisturize the baking tin, so the baking sheet sticks on it), place the tin in the oven. Lover its temperature to 180°C and bake for about 40 minutes.

Once done, the pumpkin will be fork tender.

Finally place the mixture in a blender (or pot when using submersible blender). Do not forget to free the garlic cloves from its peel. Add two cups of boiled water or veggie broth and blend it all together. Keep adding liquid to achieve the desired thickness of your soup.

Finally, you can always add more spices or salt, if you feel like the soup still needs more taste.

To mix up the recipe, replace the pumpkin with carrots or sweet potatoes. As always, be creative and have fun!

Week 4

In the final stage of the transition process you should already be used to the new eating habits you've developed. You have switched your breakfast, lunch and dinner meals to plant-based meals but the journey doesn't end there! You still have got a lot to learn, from how to combat cravings to how to make some of the most delicious plant-based meals ever! To combat your cravings, increase the intake of plant-based ingredients per meal to feel fuller and less prone to satisfy a craving. Throughout the fourth week of the program and after, you are going to be learning about new recipes that involve great plant-based meals. Learning new recipes is going to help you keep your meal plan diverse and full of nutrients. Your plant-based diet adventure does not end with this program! After the fourth week, you will be used to this type of diet but you will still have a lot to learn and a lot of material to experiment with. One very important thing to learn at this stage of the program is that you should be eating plant based, healthy snacks every day to feel fuller and reduce cravings, as well as stay energetic and productive throughout the day. Stay consistent with your meal plans and include snacks every now and then. Of course, the easiest and always go to snack should be fruit and vegetables or nuts. There is nothing easier than pull out an apple or few nuts from your bag when on the go. To make your transition smoother, make always sure you have a little snack always with you, so you don't end up eating fast food or some other processed foods. Remember you came to this world with only one body and you are not getting any other. So, you better take good care of it.

Did you have fun in the kitchen last three weeks and you feel like discovering more fun recipes, that can make your snacks more diverse and creative? Here are three great recipes for plant-based snacks!

#1 Two-Ingredients Banana- Oatmeal cookies

Ingredients:
- 1 large ripe banana
- 1 cup oats

Directions:
Simply mash the banana and mix in the oats. If desired you can still add one of following ingredients (raisins,

dried cranberries, cocoa nibs, shredded coconut, chopped nuts).

Shape tablespoons of dough on a baking sheet in a form of cookies. Bake in the oven heated on 180°C for about 10 minutes. Let them cool after taking out of the oven and enjoy.

#2 Coconut Bites

Ingredients:
- 1 cup of pineapple juice
- 2 cups of diced mango
- 2 diced ripe bananas
- ½ vanilla bean
- 4 cups of shredded coconut
- ¾ cup of toasted shredded coconut

Directions:

Use a small pot to cook the pineapple juice, bananas, mango and vanilla. Cook at low heat for five minutes. Then scrape the seeds from the vanilla bean into the pot and cook for two more minutes. Put the ingredients into the pot, process the 4 cups of shredded coconut until you have a smooth but firm mixture. Let the mixture cool down for an hour or two and then a roll small amount of it into a ball and roll it into the toasted coconut. Roll up all your coconut bites for a perfect plant-based snack!

#3 Fruit Pie

Ingredients:
- 1 cup of pitted dates
- 1 ½ cup of walnuts or pecans
- 1 tablespoon of vanilla extract
- ½ cup of shredded coconut
- ½ tablespoon of cinnamon
- Sliced fresh fruit
-

Directions:

Put all crust ingredients into a food processor and blend them until you get a paste. Press the paste into a pie pan and let it chill for a while, until it is ready to add fruit on it. Arrange the fruit on top of the pie according to your liking and cool the pie off 1 hour before serving and, voila, a perfect, healthy snack.

This plant-based diet guide was designed to introduce beginners to this kind of diet and encourage them to make the right choices regarding their eating habits. As a beginner, you don't have to feel overwhelmed and pressured by diet plans. Instead of jumping straight into it, it is more important to firstly get to know the diet and learn why it is beneficial for your health and overall well-being. That's exactly what this book was designed to do,

teach you about the plant-based diet and show you how to gradually yet surly transition to a diet without any animal products. What you should take away from this book are all the reasons why the plant-based diet positively affects your health and why it is important to manage your eating habits regularly. Upon getting to know all this information, the next step is to start implementing it in your everyday life. Ditching animal products completely sounds like a difficult task but it can actually be easy and effortless, as long as you follow the right meal plan. My plant-based diet guide will help you effortlessly transition to a plant-based diet by introducing new ingredients gradually, without pressure. Throughout this 4-week program, you will get used to plant-based ingredients and start letting go of animal products up until the point where you completely throw them out of your everyday meals. Keep in mind that diet transition is a steady process, so don't try to rush and skip steps of the meal program in hopes to achieve the results sooner. Take it easy and enjoy combining various delicious ingredients and preparing outstanding meals while receiving all the necessary nutrients for your body's proper functioning.

The Plant Based Breakfast

Chia Flaxseed Waffles

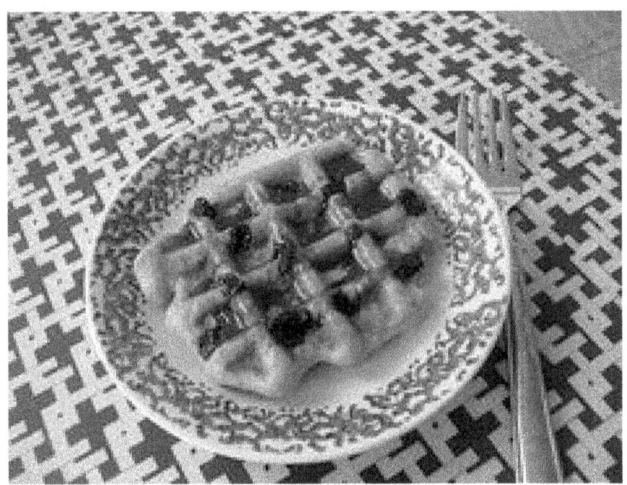

Preparation Time: 25 minutes

Servings: 8

Ingredients:

- 2 cups ground golden flaxseed
- 2 tsp cinnamon
- 10 tsp ground chia seed
- 15 tbsp warm water
- 1/3 cup coconut oil, melted

- 1/2 cup water
- 1 tbsp baking powder
- 1 tsp sea salt

Directions:
1. Preheat the waffle iron.
2. In a small bowl, mix together ground chia seed and warm water.
3. In a large bowl, mix together ground flax seed, sea salt, and baking powder. Set aside.
4. Add melted coconut oil, chia seed mixture, and water into the blender and blend for 30 seconds.
5. Transfer coconut oil mixture into the flax seed mixture and mix well. Add cinnamon and stir well.
6. Scoop waffle mixture into the hot waffle iron and cook on each side for 3-5 minutes.
7. Serve and enjoy.

Nutrition: Calories 240; Fat 20.6 g; Carbohydrates 12.9 g; Sugar 0 g; Protein 7 g; Cholesterol 0 mg;

Cauliflower Zucchini Fritters

Preparation Time: 15 minutes

Servings: 4

Ingredients:

3 cups cauliflower florets

¼ tsp black pepper

¼ cup coconut flour

2 medium zucchini, grated and squeezed

1 tbsp coconut oil

½ tsp sea salt

Directions:

Steam cauliflower florets for 5 minutes.

Add cauliflower into the food processor and process until it looks like rice.

Add all ingredients except coconut oil to the large bowl and mix until well combined.

Make small round patties from the mixture and set aside.

Heat coconut oil in a pan over medium heat.

Place patties on pan and cook for 3-4 minutes on each side.

Serve and enjoy.

Nutrition: Calories 68; Fat 3.8 g; Carbohydrates 7.8 g; Sugar 3.6 g; Protein 2.8 g; Cholesterol 0 mg;

Chocolate Strawberry Milkshake

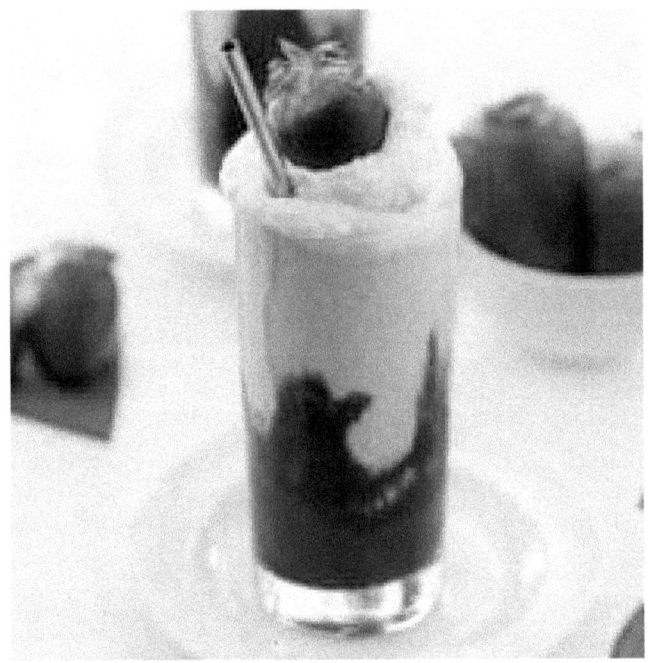

Preparation Time: 5 minutes

Servings: 2

Ingredients:

- 1 cup ice cubes
- ¼ cup unsweetened cocoa powder
- 2 scoops vegan protein powder
- 1 cup strawberries
- 2 cups unsweetened coconut milk

Directions:
1. Add all ingredients into the blender and blend until smooth and creamy.
2. Serve immediately and enjoy.

Nutrition: Calories 221; Fat 5.7 g; Carbohydrates 15 g; Sugar 6.8 g; Protein 27.7 g; Cholesterol 0 mg;

Coconut Blackberry Breakfast Bowl

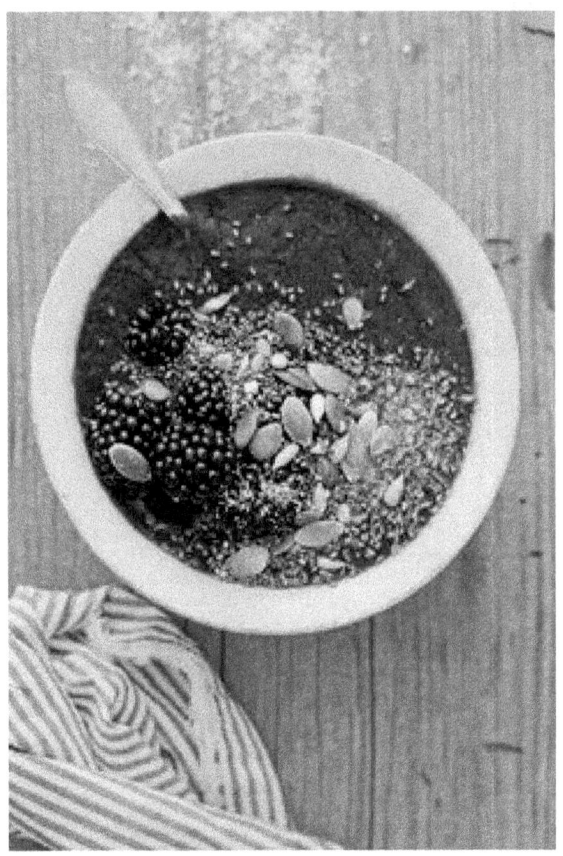

Preparation Time: 10 minutes

Servings: 2

Ingredients:

- 2 tbsp chia seeds
- ¼ cup coconut flakes

- 1 cup spinach
- ¼ cup water
- 3 tbsp ground flaxseed
- 1 cup unsweetened coconut milk
- 1 cup blackberries

Directions:

1. Add blackberries, flaxseed, spinach, and coconut milk into the blender and blend until smooth.
2. Fry coconut flakes in pan for 1-2 minutes.
3. Pour berry mixture into the serving bowls and sprinkle coconut flakes and chia seeds on top.
4. Serve immediately and enjoy.

Nutrition: Calories 182; Fat 11.4 g; Carbohydrates 14.5 g; Sugar 4.3 g; Protein 5.3 g; Cholesterol 0 mg;

Cinnamon Coconut Pancake

Preparation Time: 15 minutes

Servings: 1

Ingredients:
- 1/2 cup almond milk
- 1/4 cup coconut flour
- 2 tbsp egg replacer
- 8 tbsp water
- 1 packet stevia
- 1/8 tsp cinnamon
- 1/2 tsp baking powder
- 1 tsp vanilla extract
- 1/8 tsp salt

Directions:
1. In a small bowl, mix together egg replacer and 8 tablespoons of water.
2. Add all ingredients into the mixing bowl and stir until combined.
3. Spray pan with cooking spray and heat over medium heat.
4. Pour the desired amount of batter onto hot pan and

cook until lightly golden brown.
5. Flip pancake and cook for a few minutes more.
6. Serve and enjoy.

Nutrition: Calories 110; Fat 4.3 g; Carbohydrates 10.9 g; Sugar 2.8 g; Protein 7 g; Cholesterol 0 mg;

Flax Almond Muffins

Preparation Time: 45 minutes

Servings: 6

Ingredients:

- 1 tsp cinnamon
- 2 tbsp coconut flour
- 20 drops liquid stevia
- 1/4 cup water
- 1/4 tsp vanilla extract
- 1/4 tsp baking soda
- 1/2 tsp baking powder
- 1/4 cup almond flour
- 1/2 cup ground flax
- 2 tbsp ground chia

Directions:

1. Preheat the oven to 350 F/ 176 C.
2. Spray muffin tray with cooking spray and set aside.
3. In a small bowl, add 6 tablespoons of water and ground chia. Mix well and set aside.
4. In a mixing bowl, add ground flax, baking soda, baking powder, cinnamon, coconut flour, and

5. almond flour and mix well.
6. Add chia seed mixture, vanilla, water, and liquid stevia and stir well to combine.
7. Pour mixture into the prepared muffin tray and bake in preheated oven for 35 minutes.
8. Serve and enjoy.

Nutrition: Calories 92; Fat 6.3 g; Carbohydrates 6.9 g; Sugar 0.4 g; Protein 3.7 g; Cholesterol 0 mg;

Grain-free Overnight Oats

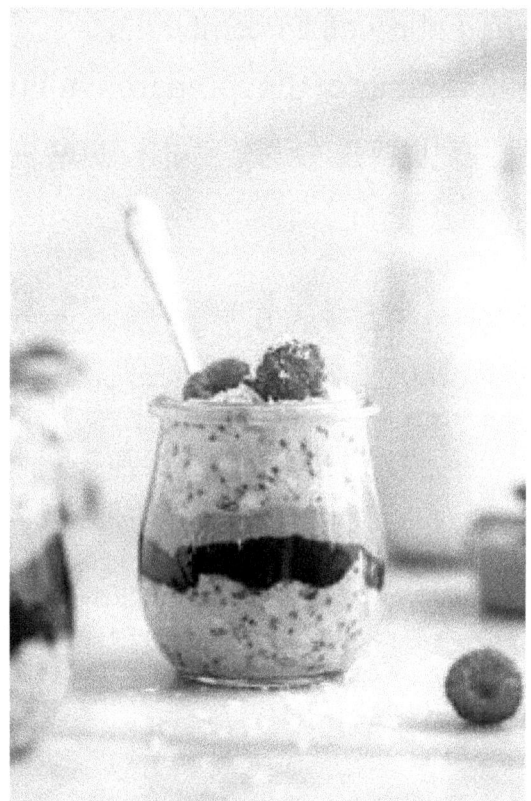

Preparation Time: 10 minutes

Servings: 1

Ingredients:

- 2/3 cup unsweetened coconut milk
- 2 tsp chia seeds
- 2 tbsp vanilla protein powder

- ½ tbsp coconut flour
- 3 tbsp hemp hearts

Directions:
1. Add all ingredients into the glass jar and stir to combine.
2. Close jar with lid and place in refrigerator for overnight.
3. Top with fresh berries and serve.

Nutrition: Calories 378; Fat 22.5 g; Carbohydrates 15 g; Sugar 1.5 g; Protein 27 g; Cholesterol 0 mg;

Zucchini Muffins

Preparation Time: 35 minutes

Servings: 8

Ingredients:
- 1 cup almond flour
- 1 zucchini, grated
- 1/4 cup coconut oil, melted
- 15 drops liquid stevia
- 1/2 tsp baking soda
- 1/2 cup coconut flour
- 1/2 cup walnut, chopped
- 1 1/2 tsp cinnamon
- 3/4 cup unsweetened applesauce
- 1/8 tsp salt

Directions:
1. Preheat the oven to 325 F/ 162 C.
2. Spray muffin tray with cooking spray and set aside.
3. In a bowl, combine together grated zucchini, coconut oil, and stevia.
4. In another bowl, mix together coconut flour, baking soda, almond flour, walnut, cinnamon, and salt.

5. Add zucchini mixture into the coconut flour mixture and mix well.
6. Add applesauce and stir until well combined.
7. Pour batter into the prepared muffin tray and bake in preheated oven for 25-30 minutes.
8. Serve and enjoy.
9.

Nutrition: Calories 229; Fat 18.9 g; Carbohydrates 12.5 g; Sugar 3.4 g; Protein 5.2 g; Cholesterol 0 mg;

Apple Avocado Coconut Smoothie

Preparation Time: 5 minutes

Servings: 2

Ingredients:

- 1 tsp coconut oil
- 1 tbsp collagen powder
- 1 tbsp fresh lime juice
- ½ cup unsweetened coconut milk
- ¼ apple, slice
- 1 avocado

Directions:

1. Add all ingredients into the blender and blend until smooth and creamy.
2. Serve and enjoy.
3.

Nutrition: Calories 262; Fat 23.9 g; Carbohydrates 13.6 g; Sugar 3.4 g; Protein 2 g; Cholesterol 0 mg;

Healthy Breakfast Granola

Preparation Time: 15 minutes

Servings: 5

Ingredients:

- 1 cup walnuts, diced
- 1 cup unsweetened coconut flakes
- 1 cup sliced almonds
- 2 tbsp coconut oil, melted
- 4 packets Splenda
- 2 tsp cinnamon

Directions:

1. Preheat the oven to 375 F/ 190 C.
2. Spray a baking tray with cooking spray and set aside.
3. Add all ingredients into the medium bowl and toss well.
4. Spread bowl mixture on a prepared baking tray and bake in preheated oven for 10 minutes.
5. Serve and enjoy.

Nutrition: Calories 458; Fat 42.5 g; Carbohydrates 13.7 g; Sugar 2.7 g; Protein 11.7 g; Cholesterol 0 mg;

Chia Cinnamon Smoothie

Preparation Time: 5 minutes

Servings: 1

Ingredients:

- 2 scoops vanilla protein powder
- 1 tbsp chia seeds
- ½ tsp cinnamon
- 1 tbsp coconut oil
- ½ cup water
- ½ cup unsweetened coconut milk

Directions:

1. Add all ingredients into the blender and blend until smooth and creamy.
2. Serve immediately and enjoy.

Nutrition: Calories 397; Fat 23.9 g; Carbohydrates 13.4 g; Sugar 0 g; Protein 31.6 g; Cholesterol 0 mg;

Vegetable Tofu Scramble

Preparation Time: 20 minutes

Servings: 2

Ingredients:

- 1 block firm tofu, drained and crumbled
- ½ tsp turmeric
- ¼ tsp garlic powder
- 1 cup spinach
- 1 red pepper, chopped
- 10 oz mushrooms, chopped
- ½ onion, chopped
- 1 tbsp olive oil
- Pepper
- Salt

Directions:

1. Heat olive oil in a large pan over medium heat.
2. Add onion, pepper, and mushrooms and sauté until cooked.
3. Add crumbled tofu, spices, and spinach. Stir well and cook for 3-5 minutes.
4. Serve and enjoy.

Nutrition: Calories 159; Fat 9.6 g; Carbohydrates 13.7 g; Sugar 7 g; Protein 9.6 g; Cholesterol 0 mg;

The Plant Based Lunch

Mac & "Cheese"

Servings: 6

Preparation Time: 40 Minutes

Calories: 848

Protein: 70 Grams

Fat: 8.4 Grams

Carbs: 140.1 Grams

Ingredients:
- Milk Substitute
- 16 Ounces Elbow Macaroni, Whole Wheat
- 16 Ounces Vegan Mayonnaise
- 3 Cups Nutritional Yeast
- Whole Wheat Bread Crumbs
- Sea Salt & Black Pepper to Taste

Directions:
1. Start by heating your oven to 350, and then make your noodles as the package instructs. Drain them,

and then add in your ingredients, and mix well.
2. Add in your milk substitute, stirring until creamy.
3. Pour your ingredients into a baking dish and then sprinkle your bread crumbs on top.

Bake until it's golden brown, which will take about a half hour.

Thai Squash Soup

Servings: 2

Preparation Time: 30 Minutes

Calories: 717.3

Protein: 10.3 Grams

Fat: 48.3 Grams

Carbs: 77.4 Grams

Ingredients:
- 1 Teaspoon Curry Powder
- 1 Tablespoon Olive Oil
- 1 Red Onion, Chopped
- 1 Pint Vegetable Stock
- 1 Butter Squash, Chunked
- 1 Can Coconut Milk (Roughly 13.5 Ounces)
-

Directions:
1. Get out a pan and heat your olive oil. Once it's heated, add in your onion and cook to soften. This should take two to three minutes. Add your butternut squash, stock to taste, and curry powder.
2. Bring it to a boil, and then reduce to simmer. The

squash should become tender.

3. Stir in your coconut milk, and then blend until smooth.
4. Return it to the pan to warm, and season with salt and pepper before serving.

Butter Bean Hummus

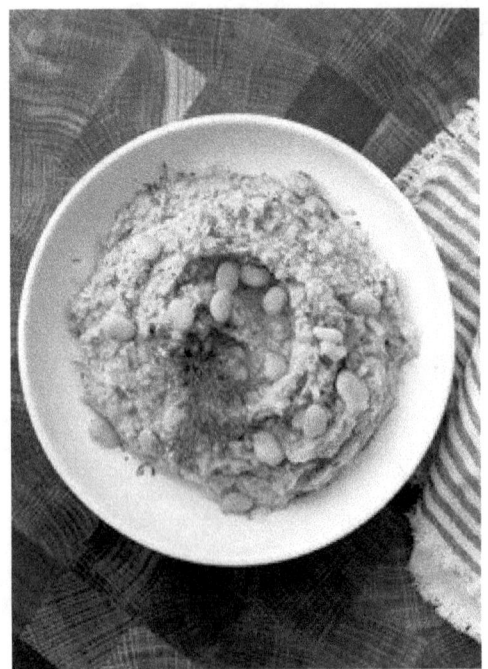

Servings: 4

Preparation Time: 5 Minutes

Calories: 150

Protein: 8 Grams

Fat: 4 Grams

Carbs: 23 Grams

Ingredients:

- 1 Can Butter Beans, Drained & Rinsed
- 4 Sprigs Parsley, Minced

- 1 Tablespoon Olive Oil
- ½ Lemon, Juiced
- 2 Cloves Garlic, Minced
- Sea Salt to Taste

Directions:

Blend all of your ingredients together, and then serve as a dip with fresh vegetables.

Spinach & Orange Salad

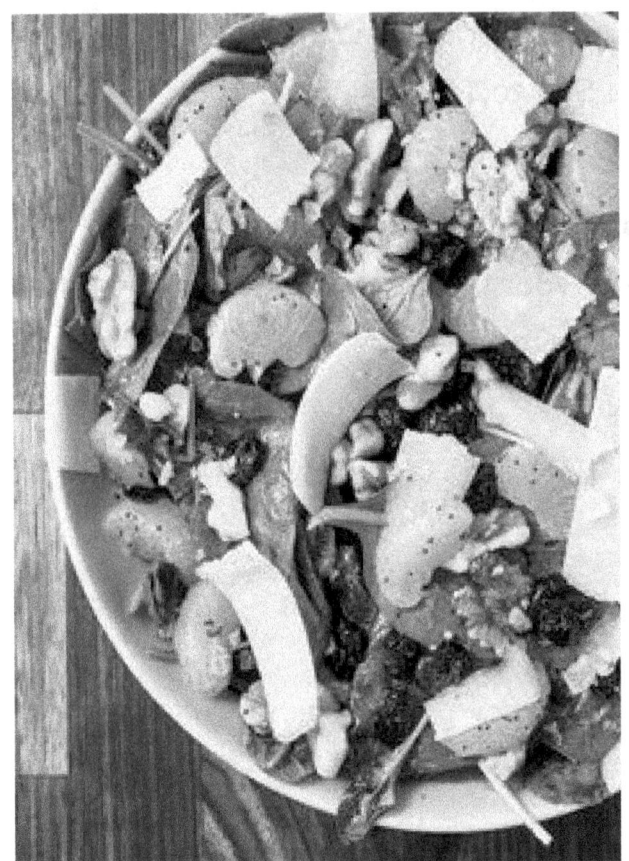

Servings: 6

Preparation Time: 15 Minutes

Calories: 99

Protein: 2.5 Grams

Fat: 5 Grams

Carbs: 13.1 Grams

Ingredients:

- ¼ -1/3 Cup Vegan Dressing
- 3 Oranges, Medium, Peeled, Seeded & Sectioned
- ¾ lb. Spinach, Fresh & Torn
- 1 Red Onion, Medium, Sliced & Separated into Rings

Directions:

Toss everything together, and serve with dressing.

Lentil & Sweet Potato Soup

Servings: 6

Preparation Time: 40 Minutes

Calories: 323

Protein: 16 Grams

Fat: 3.4 Grams

Carbs: 58.5 Grams

Ingredients:

- 1 Cup Red Lentil
- 750 Grams Sweet Potatoes
- ¼ Teaspoon Cayenne
- 3 Onions
- 1 lemon
- 5 Cloves Garlic
- ½ Teaspoon Turmeric
- ½ Cup Coriander, Chopped
- 5 Cups Water
- 2 Teaspoon Cumin
- Sea Salt & Black Pepper to Taste

Directions:

1. Start by peeling and chopping your onion and sweet potatoes, and it can be a little thick.
2. Combine your garlic, water, lentils, cumin, turmeric and cumin together in a pot.
3. Bring it to a boil, and allow it to simmer for a half hour.
4. Puree your soup before adding in your lemon juice and coriander. Season with salt and pepper to taste.

Fruity Kale Salad

Servings: 4

Preparation Time: 30 Minutes

Calories: 220

Protein: 4 Grams

Fat: 17 Grams

Carbs: 16 Grams

Ingredients:

- Salad:
- 10 Ounces Baby Kale
- ½ Cup Pomegranate Arils
- 1 Tablespoon Olive Oil
- 1 Apple, Sliced

Dressing:

- 3 Tablespoons Apple Cider Vinegar
- 3 Tablespoons Olive Oil
- 1 Tablespoon Tahini Sauce (Optional)
- Sea Salt & Black Pepper to Taste

Directions:

1. Wash and dry the kale. If kale is too expensive, you can also use lettuce, arugula or spinach. Take the stems out, and chop it.
2. Combine all of your salad ingredients together.
3. Combine all of your dressing ingredients together before drizzling it over the salad to serve.

Black Eyed Peas Stew

Servings: 5

Preparation Time: 30 Minutes

Calories: 338

Protein: 21 Grams

Fat: 4 Grams

Carbs: 58 Grams

Ingredients:

- 1 Can Tomatoes, Crushed
- ¼ Teaspoon Cayenne
- 1 Clove Garlic
- 2 Tablespoons Olive Oil
- 1 Onion
- 2 Cans Black Eyed Peas, Drained
- 8 Ounces Okra, Frozen & Thawed
- Sea Salt to Taste

Directions:

1. Start by brown your onion using olive oil, and then add in your garlic and cayenne. Cook for another minute.
2. Mix in all of your remaining ingredients, simmering until your okra becomes soft.

White Bean & Spinach Soup

Servings: 4

Preparation Time: 25 Minutes

Calories: 218

Protein: 12 Grams

Fat: 3.3 Grams

Carbs: 37.9 Grams

Ingredients:

- 3 Cups Baby Spinach, Cleaned & Trimmed
- 1 Can White Beans (Roughly 14.5 Ounces)
- 3-4 Cups Vegetable Stock, Homemade
- 1 Shallot, Diced Fine
- 1 Clove Garlic, Minced Fine
- 14.5 Ounces Tomatoes, Diced
- 1 Teaspoon Rosemary
- ½ Cup Shell Pasta, Whole Wheat
- 2 Teaspoons Olive Oil
- Red Pepper Flakes to Taste
- Black Pepper to Taste

Directions:
1. Start by heating your olive oil in a saucepan before sautéing your garlic and shallots
2. Add in your rosemary, beans, broth and tomatoes. Season with your red pepper flakes and black pepper.
3. Put your pasta in, cooking for ten minutes, and then add in your spinach. Cook until it's wilted.

Soup Salads And Sides

Mexican Cauliflower Rice

Preparation Time: 25 minutes
Servings: 4

Ingredients:

- 1 medium cauliflower head, cut into florets
- ½ cup tomato sauce
- ¼ tsp black pepper
- 1 tsp chili powder
- 2 garlic cloves, minced
- ½ medium onion, diced
- 1 tbsp coconut oil
- ½ tsp sea salt
-

Directions:

1. Add cauliflower florets into the food processor and process until it looks like rice.
2. Heat oil in a pan over medium-high heat.
3. Add onion to the pan and sauté for 5 minutes or

until softened.
4. Add garlic and cook for 1 minute.
5. Add cauliflower rice, chili powder, pepper, and salt. Stir well.
6. Add tomato sauce and cook for 5 minutes.
7. Stir well and serve warm.

Nutrition: Calories 83; Fat 3.7g; Carbohydrates 11.5 g; Sugar 5.4 g; Protein 3.6 g; Cholesterol 0 mg;

Turnip Salad

Preparation Time: 10 minutes

Servings: 4

Ingredients:

- 4 white turnips, spiralized
- 1 lemon juice
- 4 dill sprigs, chopped
- 2 tbsp olive oil
- 1 1/2 tsp salt

Directions:

1. Season spiralized turnip with salt and gently massage with hands.
2. Add lemon juice and dill. Season with pepper and salt.
3. Drizzle with olive oil and combine everything well.
4. Serve immediately and enjoy.

Nutrition: Calories 49; Fat 1.1 g; Carbohydrates 9 g; Sugar 5.2 g; Protein 1.4 g; Cholesterol 0 mg;

Brussels sprouts Salad

Preparation Time: 20 minutes
Servings: 6

Ingredients:

- 1 ½ lbs.' Brussels sprouts, trimmed
- ¼ cup toasted hazelnuts, chopped
- 2 tsp Dijon mustard
- 1 ½ tbsp lemon juice
- 2 tbsp olive oil
- Pepper
- Salt

Directions:

1. In a small bowl, whisk together oil, mustard, lemon juice, pepper, and salt.
2. In a large bowl, combine together Brussels sprouts and hazelnuts.
3. Pour dressing over salad and toss well.
4. Serve immediately and enjoy.

Nutrition: Calories 111; Fat 7.1 g; Carbohydrates 11 g; Sugar 2.7 g; Protein 4.4 g; Cholesterol 0 mg;

Tomato Eggplant Spinach Salad

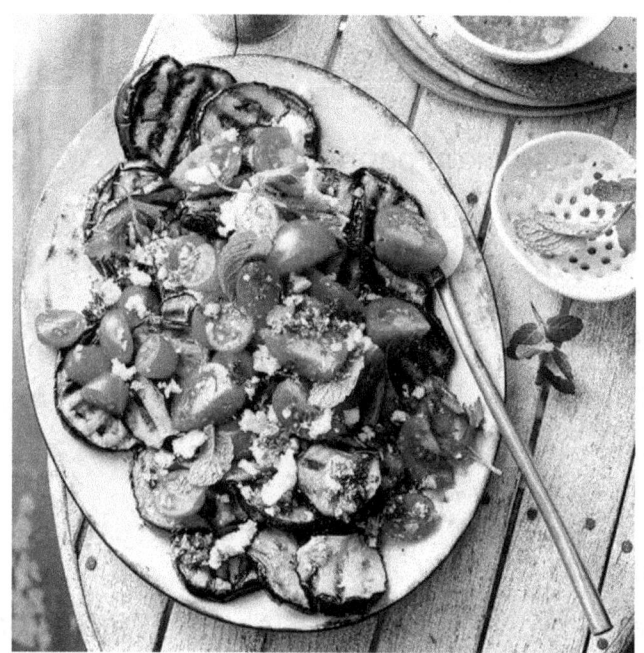

Preparation Time: 30 minutes

Servings: 4

Ingredients:

- 1 large eggplant, cut into 3/4-inch slices
- 5 oz spinach
- 1 tbsp sun-dried tomatoes, chopped
- 1 tbsp oregano, chopped
- 1 tbsp parsley, chopped

- 1 tbsp fresh mint, chopped
- 1 tbsp shallot, chopped
- For dressing:
- 1/4 cup olive oil
- 1/2 lemon juice
- 1/2 tsp smoked paprika
- 1 tsp Dijon mustard
- 1 tsp tahini
- 2 garlic cloves, minced
- Pepper
- Salt

Directions:

1. Place sliced eggplants into the large bowl and sprinkle with salt and set aside for minutes.
2. In a small bowl mix together all dressing ingredients. Set aside.
3. Heat grill to medium-high heat.
4. In a large bowl, add shallot, sun-dried tomatoes, herbs, and spinach.
5. Rinse eggplant slices and pat dry with paper towel.
6. Brush eggplant slices with olive oil and grill on medium high heat for 3-4 minutes on each side.
7. Let cool the grilled eggplant slices then cut into quarters.

8. Add eggplant to the salad bowl and pour dressing over salad. Toss well.
9. Serve and enjoy.

Nutrition: Calories 163; Fat 13 g; Carbohydrates 10 g; Sugar 3 g; Protein 2 g; Cholesterol 0 mg;

Cauliflower Radish Salad

Preparation Time: 15 minutes

Servings: 4

Ingredients:

- 12 radishes, trimmed and chopped
- 1 tsp dried dill
- 1 tsp Dijon mustard
- 1 tbsp cider vinegar
- 1 tbsp olive oil
- 1 cup parsley, chopped
- ½ medium cauliflower head, trimmed and chopped
- ½ tsp black pepper
- ¼ tsp sea salt

Directions:

1. In a mixing bowl, combine together cauliflower, parsley, and radishes.
2. In a small bowl, whisk together olive oil, dill, mustard, vinegar, pepper, and salt.
3. Pour dressing over salad and toss well.
4. Serve immediately and enjoy.

Nutrition: Calories 58; Fat 3.8 g; Carbohydrates 5.6 g; Sugar 2.1 g; Protein 2.1 g; Cholesterol 0 mg;

Celery Salad

Preparation Time: 10 minutes

Servings: 6

Ingredients:

- 6 cups celery, sliced
- ¼ tsp celery seed
- 1 tbsp lemon juice
- 2 tsp lemon zest, grated
- 1 tbsp parsley, chopped
- 1 tbsp olive oil
- Sea salt
-

Directions:

1. Add all ingredients into the large mixing bowl and toss well.
2. Serve immediately and enjoy.
3.

Nutrition: Calories 38; Fat 2.5 g; Carbohydrates 3.3 g; Sugar 1.5 g; Protein 0.8 g; Cholesterol 0 mg;

Ginger Avocado Kale Salad

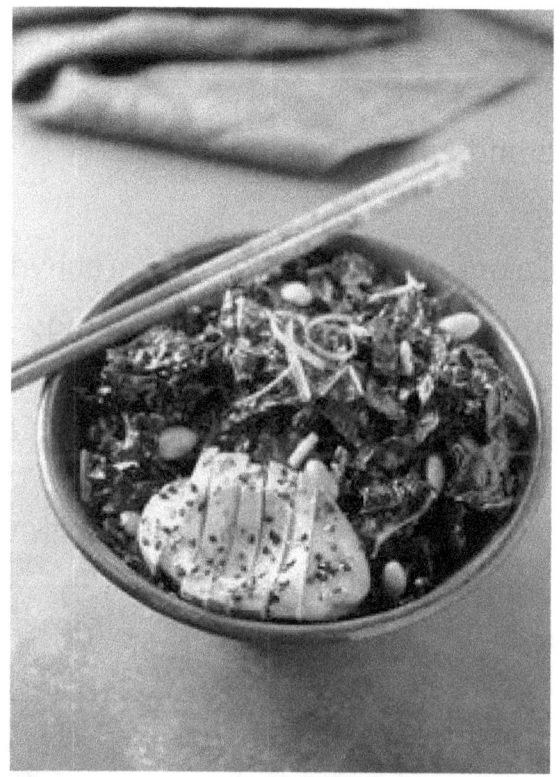

Preparation Time: 15 minutes

Servings: 4

Ingredients:

- 1 avocado, peeled and sliced
- 1 tbsp ginger, grated
- 1/2 lb. kale, chopped
- 1/4 cup parsley, chopped

- 2 fresh scallions, chopped

Directions:
1. Add all ingredients into the mixing bowl and toss well.
2. Serve and enjoy.

Nutrition: Calories 139; Fat 9.9 g; Carbohydrates 12 g; Sugar 0.5 g; Protein 3 g; Cholesterol 0 mg;

Avocado Cabbage Salad

Preparation Time: 20 minutes

Servings: 4

Ingredients:

- 2 avocados, diced
- 4 cups cabbage, shredded
- 3 tbsp fresh parsley, chopped
- 2 tbsp apple cider vinegar
- 4 tbsp olive oil
- 1 cup cherry tomatoes, halved
- 1/2 tsp pepper
- 1 1/2 tsp sea salt
-

Directions:

1. Add cabbage, avocados, and tomatoes to a medium bowl and mix well.
2. In a small bowl, whisk together oil, parsley, vinegar, pepper, and salt.
3. Pour dressing over vegetables and mix well.
4. Serve and enjoy.

Nutrition: Calories 253; Fat 21.6 g; Carbohydrates 14 g; Sugar 4 g; Protein 3.5 g; Cholesterol 0 mg;

Vegetable Salad

Preparation Time: 15 minutes

Servings: 6

Ingredients:
- 2 cups cauliflower florets
- 2 cups carrots, chopped
- 2 cups cherry tomatoes, halved
- 2 tbsp shallots, minced
- 1 bell pepper, seeded and chopped
- 1 cucumber, seeded and chopped

For dressing:
- 2 garlic cloves, minced
- 1/2 cup red wine vinegar
- 1/2 cup olive oil
- Pepper
- Salt

Directions:
1. In a small bowl, combine together all dressing ingredients.
2. Add all salad ingredients to the large bowl and toss

well.
3. Pour dressing over salad and toss well.
4. Place salad bowl in refrigerator for 4 hours.
5. Serve chilled and enjoy.

Nutrition: Calories 200; Fat 17.1 g; Carbohydrates 12.1 g; Sugar 6.1 g; Protein 2.2 g; Cholesterol 0 mg;

Refreshing Cucumber Salad

Preparation Time: 10 minutes

Servings: 4

Ingredients:
- 1/3 cup cucumber basil ranch
- 1 cucumber, chopped
- 3 tomatoes, chopped
- 3 tbsp fresh herbs, chopped
- ½ onion, sliced

Directions:
1. Add all ingredients into the large mixing bowl and toss well.
2. Serve immediately and enjoy.

Nutrition: Calories 84; Fat 3.4 g; Carbohydrates 12.5 g; Sugar 6.8 g; Protein 2 g; Cholesterol 0 mg;

Avocado Almond Cabbage Salad

Preparation Time: 15 minutes

Servings: 3

Ingredients:

- 3 cups savoy cabbage, shredded
- ½ cup blanched almonds
- 1 avocado, chopped
- ¼ tsp pepper
- ¼ tsp sea salt
- For dressing:
- 1 tsp coconut aminos
- ½ tsp Dijon mustard
- 1 tbsp lemon juice
- 3 tbsp olive oil
- Pepper
- Salt

Directions:

1. In a small bowl, mix together all dressing ingredients and set aside.
2. Add all salad ingredients to the large bowl and mix well.

3. Pour dressing over salad and toss well.
4. Serve immediately and enjoy.

Nutrition: Calories 317; Fat 14.1 g; Carbohydrates 39.8 g; Sugar 9.3 g; Protein 11.6 g; Cholesterol 0 mg;

www.ingramcontent.com/pod-product-compliance
Lightning Source LLC
Chambersburg PA
CBHW070722030426
42336CB00013B/1895